BREASTFEEDING

The Essential Guide for

New Parents and Carers

EVE WINTERS

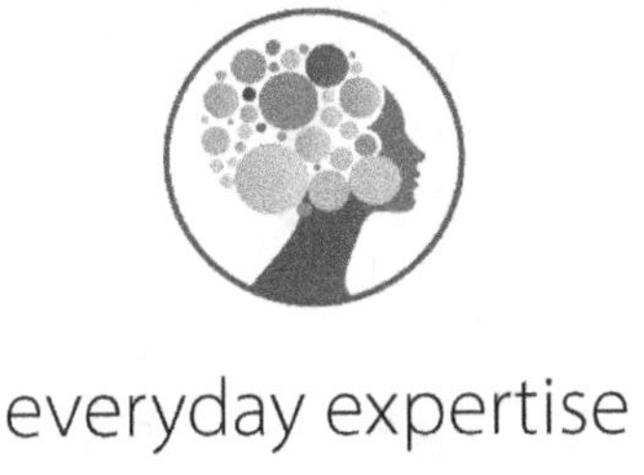

everyday expertise

BREASTFEEDING

The Essential Guide for

New Parents and Carers

Foreword

Like most children of the 1970s I was exclusively bottle-fed on government-provided formula. In fact, my parents' attitude to breastfeeding could be best summed up as "ick" and in this they were entirely in tune with the thinking of the day. By the time I had my own babies in in the noughties, however, there had been a complete change in public health messaging. Suddenly "breast was best" and midwives and health visitors provided leaflets and motivational talks about why to breastfeed.

As a result, I was determined to breastfeed – of course, I wanted the best for my baby. But breastfeeding is not as easy as those leaflets suggested nor did the pro-breastfeeding talks I attended before going into labour in any way to reflect the level of support available once there was an actual howling and hungry baby in my arms. Of the six women on my maternity ward, I was the only one who chose to breastfeed, and the over-stretched midwives made me feel like a nuisance when I asked for help getting baby into the right position. And of the 10 women I'd met in my pre-natal classes, only me and one other mum, a nurse herself, breastfed. "Breast may be best" but for me, and many other women, there wasn't support where it mattered, in those first hours, days and weeks after birth. I was largely left to work things out for myself and there followed a lot of sleepless nights, tears (both me and baby) and sore boobs. But somehow we figured it out and in the end, I breastfed three babies, one for six months, one for 10 months and one for almost two years (always the littlest, huh?).

If you're thinking about breastfeeding or are struggling right now with the practicalities, then I hope this book provides some useful advice and insight to help you and baby find your way forward.

Breastfeeding is a remarkable gift: you are feeding a fast-growing brand-new human being with nothing but the outputs of your own body. But it's important to keep perspective. Breastmilk is not the only way to nourish and bond with your newborn. However you feed your baby, you're embarking on a journey of love, growth and bonding that will last a lifetime.

1.   Why breastfeed

Breastfeeding is a feeding system that is portable, available 24/7, a proven immune-booster and nutritional superfood, and it's free. It's amazing it was ever replaced but in the middle of the 20th century formula milk was positioned as the convenient, clean, modern and nutritional equivalent that could release women from the "tyranny" of being solely responsible for feeding. Those decades saw the loss of much maternal knowledge, which means when public health agencies once again decided to promote breastfeeding there wasn't a cultural and societal support base for lactating mothers and the knowhow to help get started right was lacking. And, with breastfeeding, the early days really are key.

Although it varies from country to country, and region to region, in many developed countries as many as 80% or more of mothers will attempt breastfeeding in the hospital or shortly after birth. But this proportion very quickly falls, with many introducing mixed feeding or switching to an exclusive formula diet within weeks.

The World Health Organization's official advice is for babies to be fed only breast milk (without any formula or other liquids or solids) for the first six months. However, social pressures, the need to go out to work and general exhaustion mean this target is often missed. No-one should ever feel guilty about this – your baby will grow and thrive and love you whether fed breastmilk or formula milk. Everyone must do what is right for them, and their family. Weighing the costs In an ideal world, money would not be a consideration when deciding how to feed our babies. But in the real world, we have to acknowledge there are different costs and trade-offs to make including the high costs of formula, particularly if a baby has digestive issues or allergies, and the practicalities of mothers returning to work.

Formula: The costs vary by brand. According to the Office of the US Surgeon General, families who follow best breastfeeding advice can save between $1,200 and $1,500 in expenditures on formula in the first year alone[1]. To this, there is also the cost of bottles, teats (or nipples as they're called in North America) and sterilising equipment, which can add up over time. On the other hand, it may be easier for mothers to return to work earlier than their breastfeeding counterparts, improving family income and career prospects (albeit this may add childcare costs, which can be very expensive in some areas).

Breastfeeding: The milk is free but there are indirect costs: nursing bras and pads, breast pump, bottles and sterilising equipment. There are also potentially lost earnings if a mother decides to stay home longer in order to devote more time to breastfeeding.

2. Benefits of breastfeeding

Breastfeeding is one of those wonderfully symbiotic activities that we often find in nature, with benefits to both mother and baby. This isn't Earth Mother talk, it's established science that breastmilk has measurable health benefits for both. Let's take a look at the benefits for baby:

An all-in-one food. Breast milk is considered the gold standard for infant nutrition. It contains the perfect balance of nutrients, including proteins, fats, carbohydrates, vitamins, and minerals, tailored to the baby's needs.

Immune System Support. Your baby's immune system is booting up to learn about all about this brand-new world they have just arrived in. Breast milk is like a primer, coding information from your developed immune system to give your baby a heads up on what to expect. Rich in antibodies, enzymes, and white blood cells, this food can help protect baby against respiratory, ear and gastrointestinal infections. In fact, when your baby is unwell their spit will communicate this fact to the cells in your breast, sending a message to your immune system to increase the number of leukocytes (a type of white blood cell) in the breast milk to protect baby. Amazing!

Gut health. Breast milk is easily digested, reducing the likelihood of constipation and diarrhoea in infants. It is also less likely to cause allergies or intolerances compared to formula, which is typically derived from cow's milk.

Brain development. Breast milk contains essential fatty acids like DHA and ARA, which are crucial for brain and eye development.

Reduces the Risk of Chronic Diseases: Breastfeeding has been linked to a decreased risk of various chronic conditions in later life, including obesity, type 2 diabetes, and certain autoimmune diseases.

SIDS Prevention: Exclusive breastfeeding for the first six months of life has been associated with a reduced risk of sudden infant death syndrome (SIDS).

And for the mother

Postpartum Recovery. Breastfeeding stimulates uterine contractions, helping the mother's uterus return to its normal size more quickly and reducing postpartum bleeding. This isn't about slipping back into your pre-pregnancy jeans but about the recovery from nine-months of major biological change not to mention the intense experience of giving birth.

Contraceptive effect. Exclusive breastfeeding can act as a natural form of birth control in the early postpartum period, but it is not foolproof – there are plenty of humans walking around today as a result of parents who relied too heavily on breastfeeding's contraceptive effect!

Weight Loss. Breastfeeding burns extra calories, which can help mothers shed pregnancy weight more easily. But, as with breastfeeding's contraceptive effects, this is not a given: breastfeeding can also make you crave sugary foods and, if your breasts are uncomfortably full or you're tired from cluster feeding, you may be less inclined to exercise. As with all things in life, you need to find a balance that works for you.

Reduced Risk of Breast and Ovarian Cancer. Breastfeeding is associated with a lower risk of breast and ovarian cancers in mothers.

Emotional Well-being. Breastfeeding can release hormones like oxytocin, which promote relaxation and emotional well-being, reducing stress and postpartum depression risk.

Bonding that lasts a lifetime

There's always a lot of talk about the emotional bond that's forged when a mother breastfeeds her child. The imagery is very potent, of mother and child gazing with devotion at one another as the mother nourishes her growing infant. Yet the same is true for formula-fed babies – what matters is the comfort, eye contact, and nourishment, all of which can be given when bottle-feeding. Skin-to-skin contact, which is so important to newborn babies, can be given when formula-feeding — and using a bottle allows dads and other care givers to get in on the act. As always, it's important to do what is right for you and your family.

Why is skin-to-skin so important?

Sometimes known as kangaroo care, skin-to-skin is incredibly important for newborn babies. It helps not just by steadying their emotions but also in delivering real physiological benefits.

Regulation of Body Temperature. A newborn baby's ability to regulate body temperature is still developing. Skin-to-skin contact helps to stabilize their temperature by using the mother's body as a source of warmth and comfort.

Stabilizing Heart Rate and Breathing. Skin-to-skin contact has been shown to help regulate a baby's heart rate and breathing patterns.

Promoting Bonding and Attachment. Physical contact with the mother or primary caregiver in the form of skin-to-skin care fosters a strong emotional bond and attachment between the baby and caregiver.

Reducing Stress and Crying. Skin-to-skin contact is soothing for newborns and helps reduce their stress levels. Babies held close to their caregiver cry less and feel more secure.

Pain Relief. Skin-to-skin contact can provide natural pain relief for newborns. The mother's touch and warmth have been shown to reduce the perception of pain in babies, making medical procedures less distressing.

Improved Sleep Patterns. Babies who experience kangaroo care often have more organized sleep patterns. The closeness to the mother's body helps regulate their sleep-wake cycle.

Boosting Milk Production. For breastfeeding mothers, skin-to-skin contact can stimulate the release of oxytocin, which plays an important role in milk production and letdown.

Support for Premature and Low Birth Weight Babies. Kangaroo care is particularly beneficial for premature and low birth weight infants. It can help with weight gain, temperature regulation, and overall well-being.

Promoting Parental Confidence and Emotional Wellbeing.
Skin-to-skin contact helps build a strong sense of confidence and competence in parents, especially in the early days of caring for a newborn. It also enhances their feelings of closeness and connection with their baby, reducing stress and promoting overall well-being.

Maximising skin-to-skin

Breastfeeding has skin-to-skin and all of its amazing benefits built-in as a standard feature. Make the very most of these by wearing loose fitting, easy access nightdress or robe (this will be handy for air-drying your nipples to prevent soreness and cracking). Then get comfortable, strip baby down to nappy and allow them to snuggle up to your bare skin. If it's chilly, use a shawl or light blanket so you don't get cold. Schedule snuggle time. Life is busy, particularly if you're also juggling older children and a job. But set time aside for some quiet periods in the day, perhaps early morning or the post-bath routine where you and baby can snuggle warm skin to warm skin.

Boost bonding time by switching off all other distractions for a while. Silence the phone, switch off the TV and give your toddler a distracting activity for fifteen minutes. Look down at your baby, connect with their eyes (unless they're already blissed out and getting ready to doze), stroke a finger over their head, or hold a tiny finger.

You may be exhausted and sore and full of worries but in the grand scheme of life these moments are fleeting. Give in to the moment, feel the love and be proud of what you did: you built a human and are nourishing their body and soul for the great adventure of life that lies ahead.

3.   The science of

breastfeeding

This book is purposefully short because you'll never be busier than these crazy baby days. We're here to give you a brief lowdown so you can breastfeed with confidence, troubleshoot any issues and get on with living your best life.

But sometimes, because we're nerds at heart, it's good to know a bit of the science so you understand your body better and how the wondrous act of breastfeeding is actually a two-person job between you and your baby.

Some basics

During pregnancy your body is already busy preparing to feed your baby through a complex interplay of hormones. This is done through two hormones, prolactin and oxytocin.

During pregnancy, the placenta produces high levels of oestrogen and progesterone, which inhibit the action of prolactin, which is often referred to as the "milk-making hormone" because it plays a central role in stimulating milk production in the mammary glands of the breast. This hormonal balance prevents the mother from producing milk during pregnancy.

After childbirth, when the placenta is delivered, there is a sharp drop in progesterone levels, which allows prolactin to become active. But the hormone alone isn't enough to produce milk. It is the action of your baby suckling and the sensation of the nipple being stimulated that send signals to the mother's brain to release prolactin. Prolactin then travels through the bloodstream to the mammary glands, where it prompts milk production.

Prolactin production is directly related to the frequency and effectiveness of breastfeeding. The more a baby nurses, the more prolactin is produced, which, in turn, stimulates more milk production. This establishes a supply-and-demand system to meet the baby's needs. You may find in the early days of breastfeeding your baby is feeding like an insatiable beast and you will doubt your ability to satisfy your baby and retain your sanity – don't worry, this will be a temporary phase as your baby sends signals to your brain to release more milk. If you weren't so tired, you would realise what an amazing interplay this is!

The other important hormone is oxytocin, the "let-down hormone" because it is responsible for the release of milk from the mammary glands. It's an amazing hormone too because it is released not just in response to the sensation of the baby suckling but also if you hear your baby (sometimes any baby) crying or even just think about your baby.

When oxytocin is released, it causes the muscles surrounding the milk-filled alveoli in the breast to contract. This contraction pushes the milk down the milk ducts and out through the nipple, making it available for the baby to consume. You may be surprised to know that milk doesn't come out through a single hole like a faucet but through a series of holes (more like a shower head) which is why you might sometimes be surprised by a squirt of milk in the wrong direction!

But did you know oxytocin isn't just responsible for the release of milk? It also has an important role in regulating the mother's mood, fostering feelings of relaxation, contentment and helping build those feelings of love and attachment that are associated with breastfeeding. This dynamic system of prolactin, oxytocin and your baby's suckling ensures your body produces and delivers the right amount of milk at the right time to nourish the needs of your growing infant. It also promotes feelings of love and contentment that encourage you to sit and gaze at your new baby, spending enough time to fully establish your milk supply and encourage bonding so you will protect your offspring. Nature truly is amazing.

What is breastmilk?

Almost everything we eat and drink comes with a nutritional information label attached. But with breastmilk, you're taking it on trust that your body knows best, right? Well not quite, because scientists have spent many years studying and understanding breastmilk and what makes it such a super superfood. And breastmilk isn't just breastmilk: it comes in many guises to give your baby what they need when they need it.

Colostrum comes first…

Sometimes known as liquid gold because it is so rich in nutrients and immune protection and tends to have a yellowish colour - is produced in small quantities just before and after birth. It also has a mild laxative effect, which helps your newborn pass meconium, the thick, sticky, dark-green or black stool that accumulates in their intestines during pregnancy and makes those first newborn nappies so challenging. Colostrum also contains enzymes that help your baby's immature digestive system break down and absorb nutrients from milk and other early feeds, helps promote beneficial gut bacteria and growth factors to help your baby's earliest development.

I have known mothers who, for a variety of personal reasons didn't want to breastfeed but they still collected the colostrum to give to their babies because it's such a potent immune booster. This can be done just by firmly pressing on the breast after birth (you may want to get a midwife or birth partner to help) and collecting the liquid in a sterilized milk cup so it can be added to those first bottle feeds.

…then your milk production kicks in

After a few days the colostrum stops and your milk flow will have a different composition, produced in more substantial quantities to meet the growing baby's needs. It is mainly made up of water, proteins, lipids (fats) and lactose (carbohydrates) along with all the good stuff such as immunoglobulins and antibodies, vitamins, minerals and enzymes. All these goodies don't come out in one uniform stream of milk but are instead separated into foremilk and hindmilk.

Foremilk is released at the beginning of a feeding session and is relatively lower in fat content but higher in lactose.

Hindmilk is produced later in the feeding session and has a higher fat content. It's often richer and creamier, providing more calories and helping the baby feel full and satisfied.

This is why it's important to let your baby take their time feeding so they fully drain the breast and get all the goodness they need to grow and thrive.

A thirst-quencher too

Your breastmilk is composed of everything your baby needs for hydration and nutrition. For exclusively breastfed babies during the first six months of life[2], it is generally not necessary to provide additional water – after all, breast milk is more than 80% water[3], and it provides all the hydration a healthy term infant needs in the early months of life, even in hot or dry climates.

Your breastmilk is adapted in composition to provide more watery milk at the beginning of a feed to quench the baby's thirst, with the richer hindmilk following later in the feed. You can check your baby is well-hydrated by the frequency and colour of their wet nappies.

Giving water to a breastfed baby during the first six months can lead to overhydration and the baby may fill up on water and breastfeed less, potentially reducing milk supply. If the water is unclean, there is also the risk of passing on gastrointestinal infections.

But there are occasions when water might be needed, perhaps during extremely hot weather or if there's a risk of dehydration due to illness. In such cases, it's essential to consult with a healthcare provider for guidance.

After six months, when baby is weaning and being introduced to solid foods, then you should offer small sips of water in addition to breastmilk. However, for young babies breastmilk will continue to be the primary source of nutrition and hydration for some time.

4.   Getting ready

Well done, just by reading this far you're already well on your way to being an Everyday Expert in Breastfeeding. As you will see, breastfeeding is a wondrous interplay between a woman's hormones and her baby, delivering all the nourishment an infant needs to grow and develop.

Now let's get down to some of the practical stuff

First, in the final months of pregnancy your breasts will become heavier. It's time to invest in a good support bra for comfort and support and think about a nursing bra that will allow you to feed discreetly once baby arrives. This is also the time to buy some nursing pads to slip inside the cup of your bra because you may find as your baby's arrival gets closer that your breasts leak a little colostrum. This is normal. Colostrum is a pre-milk liquid that is rich in antibodies and essential nutrients and is an ideal first food for a newborn.

Now, it may seem that breastfeeding is the most natural thing in the world and you need do nothing to prepare. This may be true for some but actually it's a learned skill for both mother and baby. Some babies are naturals, others it takes a little time to get the action right. And for mums raised in a society where bottle-feeding has been the norm and breasts are celebrated for titillation or covered in shame, it's going to take some practice to learn this lost art. The good news is that we've got you covered, and you'll soon be an everyday expert!

Knowledge is power. Many hospitals and health clinics run classes, in person or online, where you can learn about breastfeeding techniques, latch-on methods, and common challenges. Speak to mums who have breastfed their children to get their top tips but don't allow other people's horror stories put you off. As with birth, there seems to be a human propensity to share and exaggerate bad news, but their experience isn't yours. Learn what you can but don't overthink it.

Build a Support System. Find out whether there are lactation support services in your area and work out where there are breastfeeding friendly cafes and playgroups. Having a network of experts and like-minded mothers can be invaluable in those early weeks and months.

Create a Comfortable Space. Designate a cozy and peaceful nook for breastfeeding at home. A comfortable chair, soft pillows, dim lighting and a handy table for a glass of water or muslin cloth can make all the difference.

Tell your midwife your plans. Make sure your healthcare provider knows you want to breastfeed so they can help you after birth. Even if you have a C-Section, whether planned or emergency, you can still do skin-to-skin post-delivery as this is when the magic begins.

Baby's milk-seeking instincts

Your baby is born with an inbuilt GPS system that guides them towards the safety and sustenance of their mother's breast. The newborn crawling reflex, also known as the breast crawl, kicks in shortly after birth when the baby is placed skin-to-skin on their mother's chest and uses a keen sense of smell to find their way to the breast. My first born was a difficult birth which led to a scary emergency C-Section but when the little pink nine-pounder was placed on my chest in the recovery room, where I was still reeling from the events of the previous 48 hours, I was amazed to see her shuffle about and snuffle her way up to my breast. She knew what to do even if I was still in shock!

When your newborn reaches the breast – possibly with or without your intervention - they will begin to nuzzle and "root". "Rooting" is an instinctive response that helps the baby find and latch onto their mother's breast or a bottle to feed. It is triggered when a baby's cheek or mouth is touched or brushed lightly, perhaps by your finger or nipple. When the baby feels this touch, they turn their head towards the source of the stimulus and start to open their mouth and make sucking movements. Once the baby finds the nipple or bottle, they will latch onto it and begin to suckle to get the nourishment they seek. It's an important survival mechanism because it helps newborns – who are pretty helpless compared to most species – locate a source of food and initiate feeding. As your baby develops more head and body control, the rooting reflex will diminish.

Recognising rooting behaviours – and other hunger cues, such as chewing on their fist - is a great way to anticipate when your baby is hungry so you can avert a full-blown meltdown. If your baby is a poor feeder, knowing how to stimulate rooting – by gently stroking their face – can help them feed more regularly.

Checklist

Comfortable, easy access tops. You can buy specialist breastfeeding tops and dresses, which have discreet panels and flaps to make it quick and easy to breastfeed. But this can get expensive. Any button-open blouse or shirt will do – just keep a muslin cloth or lightweight scarf to drape over your breast and baby's head if you want to protect your modesty or create a quiet den while baby feeds. Tuck it into the shoulder strap of your bra to secure it and then let it hang loosely over your chest.

Nursing bra. A good nursing bra makes a big difference. Buy a couple as you will need to wash them regularly due to leakage and those post-birth sweats

Breast pads. These can be very useful to protect your bra and cloths from embarrassing leaks.

Lanolin-based nipple ointment. This not only helps protect your nipple from the rigours of a hungry baby's suckling but also promotes healing should you be sore.

Muslin cloths. Have a good supply for soaking up mess (breastfed babies sick up less than formula-fed babies but it still happens) and as a handy modesty cover when feeding.

Pillows. You can buy all sorts of fancy breastfeeding pillows, but your normal bedroom ones will do to prop you up, support baby or protect a C-Section scar. You will become an expert at finding the right position and arrangement for you. I did find a pregnancy pillow (a sort of long squashy pillow that helped me sleep in those final uncomfortable months of pregnancy) doubled as a great breastfeeding support.

Nursing chair. You can buy specialist breastfeeding chairs that quietly glide and have arm rests well suited to breastfeeding but really any quiet corner, be it your bed or a comfortable chair will do.

Breast pump and bottles. Even if you plan on exclusive breastfeeding and staying home with baby, it can make sense to buy a basic pump and bottles/cups. Life never goes as planned and sometimes you may need to be away from baby – for medical appointments, for example.

Breastmilk containers. You can buy special containers or breastmilk storage bags for storing and freezing extra milk.

Sterilising equipment. After washing in hot soapy water, you can soak the equipment in special sterilising fluid available in all supermarkets or buy a steam steriliser – this is useful is you are planning to do a lot of expressing and bottle-feeding.

Selecting the right nursing bra

Wait Until Your Breasts Change. Your breast size can change significantly during pregnancy and after childbirth. It's a good idea to wait until closer to your due date or until your milk supply has stabilized (usually a few weeks postpartum) before buying nursing bras to ensure a better fit.

Easy Access. Look for bras with easy, one-handed access for nursing. Drop-down cups, clips, or clasps should be simple to use, especially when you have a hungry baby in your arms.

Support. The band and shoulder straps should be wide to reduce the pressure and provide comfort and support. The band should be snug but not overly tight.

Comfortable Fabric. Choose a nursing bra made of soft, breathable, and stretchy fabric. Look for options that wick away moisture to keep you dry and comfortable.

Multiple Bras. It's a good idea to have a few nursing bras on hand, including at least one sleep bra for nighttime comfort and one or two regular bras for daily wear.

Budget Considerations. Nursing bras come in a range of price points so do shop around. Look online for mums who are selling on their stock – many will be in great condition and a fraction of the price of new.

5. The three-point plan to success

Successful breastfeeding depends on three things:

- **The right position**
- **The right latch**
- **The frequency of feeding**

The right position

Experiment with different breastfeeding positions to discover what's most comfortable for both you and your baby. The popular image of a baby cradled in the mother's arms isn't necessarily going to be right for you and your baby. Many breastfeeding mums actually find the "football hold" and "side-lying" to be more comfortable for them.

Let's break these down.

Cradle Hold. The classic position, with the baby's head in the crook of your arm (the same side as the breast you're nursing from) with their body facing yours tummy to tummy. Your baby's mouth should align with your nipple, and you can use the other arm to support your breast and your baby's body. It can help to put a cushion under the baby to help support their weight, particularly as they get heavier or if you're recovering from a C-Section.

Football Hold (Clutch Hold). In this position, your baby is tucked under your arm on the same side as the breast you're nursing from, with their legs and body positioned beside you. Your hand supports their head, and you guide them to your breast. This position can be helpful if you've had a C-Section or have larger breasts.

Side-Lying Position. Lie down on your side with your baby facing you. Your baby's head should be at breast level, and they can latch onto your breast from the side. This position can be comfortable for nighttime feedings or when you want to rest while nursing.

Upright or Koala Hold. Hold your baby in an upright position, with their chest against yours. This position can be helpful if your baby has reflux or if you want to encourage a strong latch.

Twin Nursing. When breastfeeding twins, you can use different combinations of the above positions, such as double football hold or tandem cradle hold, to feed both babies simultaneously.

The right latch

The latch is how your baby attaches to your breast. When your baby breastfeeds, they are not just sucking at your nipple – they need to take a good mouthful of nipple, areola (the dark area around the nipple) and breast tissue in order to properly stimulate the milk glands and release the production of milk.

Hold Your Baby Close. Bring your baby to your breast, keeping their body close to yours. Ensure their entire body, including their head and neck, is aligned with their hips so they are not uncomfortably twisted to feed. If you are in cradle hold, a good tip is to align tummy-to-tummy, so they are turned to face you.

Big and wide. Position your baby so that their nose is aligned with your nipple. This encourages them to open their mouth wide, so they can take in more breast tissue. Wait until they open up wide before letting them latch on: their chin should touch your breast and their lips should firm a wide seal around the areola. The lips should be flanged out like a fish, not tucked in. Make sure your baby's tongue extends over their lower gumline to prevent nipple compression and discomfort.

If your baby doesn't open up wide, they may just suck on your nipple, causing pain and discomfort for you and frustration for a hungry baby. If you feel they haven't latched on right, break the latch by inserting your little finger into the baby's mouth to break the seal, and then try again. Be patient, it's better to get it right than to rush it and suffer with painful nipples.

Listen for Swallowing. You should hear your baby swallow during breastfeeding. Swallowing indicates that they are getting milk. Watch for rhythmic, deep jaw movements as your baby feeds. These movements should be slow and coordinated.

Burping. After feeding on one breast, burp your baby before switching to the other breast. Hold your baby over your shoulder and pat firmly on their back. Have a muslin cloth ready for any spit up.

One breast, then the next. After feeding on one side, and having a little winding session, offer baby the second breast so they can feed more if they wish. You may find baby isn't hungry or falls asleep before draining the second breast, in which case be sure to offer this breast first next time (or use a breast pump to fully drain the milk). In the haze of sleepless nights, you might find you lose track – with my first baby, I found it handy to keep a chart of which breast she fed from first, and the length of each feed as it helped me understand how much she was feeding and whether she was really crying for milk or could it be something else?

Visit www.everydayexpertise.net for a FREE chart to help track your baby's feeding routine.

Seek Help. If you're having difficulty achieving a correct latch, consider seeking guidance from a lactation consultant or a healthcare provider. They can provide personalized assistance and recommendations.

Frequency of feeding

Breastfeeding is a dynamic system between mother and baby. The more your baby feeds, the more milk your body produces to meet their growing needs. In the early days, it may feel like your baby is never off your breast – this is because your baby, who only has a small stomach, is striving to meet their voracious energy needs and sending signals to your body to ramp up milk production.

Newborns (0-1 month) should be breastfed on demand. Don't attempt to introduce any kind of schedule. Follow your baby's hunger cues – such as rooting, sucking on firsts or crying – and respond to them. This gives you the best chance of establishing an abundant milk supply for the weeks and months ahead. The frequency may be every two to three hours, or sometimes even more frequently, particularly when the baby is "cluster feeding".

Yes, it can be exhausting so try to sleep when baby sleeps and muster support from friends and family to help with other duties and provide you with nutritious food and drinks.

Again, in the haze of disrupted sleep, it can be helpful to keep track of feeds to work out why baby is crying and understand your baby's needs.

Visit www.everydayexpertise.net for a FREE chart to help track your baby's feeding routine.

1-2 months: As your baby grows and their stomach capacity increases, they may start to go slightly longer between feeds, but they still require frequent feedings. Feeding on demand remains important during this stage.

2-6 months: Many babies settle into a more predictable feeding routine, with feedings occurring every 2-4 hours during the day. Nighttime feedings may still be needed, but some babies may start to sleep for longer stretches at night.

6 months and beyond: As your baby begins to incorporate solid foods into their diet, the frequency of breastfeeding may decrease slightly. However, breast milk or formula should still be a significant part of their nutrition until at least 12 months of age. The exact feeding schedule can vary greatly among babies, but you can continue to breastfeed on demand and offer breast milk before or after solid meals.

These are general guidelines, and every baby is unique. Some babies may need more frequent feedings, while others may naturally go longer between feeds. The frequency of feeds can change during growth spurts, teething, illness, and other factors. Trust your instincts, follow your baby's lead and check-in regularly with your health visitor or paediatrician to make sure baby's growth is on track.

Remember, breastfeeding is not just about nourishment; it's also a way for your baby to seek comfort and bonding with you. Sometimes baby may be seeking the comfort of being cradled rather than being hungry – and that's OK too.

Cluster feeding

Cluster feeding is a period where baby feeds more frequently and often in shorter bursts over a relatively short period, such as a few hours. It can be exhausting and prompt concerns that you're not producing enough milk, but this is actually a normal behaviour among breastfeeding infants, serving several purposes:

Calorie Intake. Babies may cluster feed to increase their calorie intake in preparation for a longer sleep stretch during the night. By taking in more milk in the evening, they may be able to sleep for longer stretches without waking up hungry. I certainly noticed a period of exhausting cluster feeding would be followed by a sudden growth spurt – in hindsight it made sense but at the time I was frustrated and exhausted by this apparent backwards step.

Breast Milk Supply. Cluster feeding can stimulate the mother's breasts to produce more milk in response to the baby's growing needs.

Comfort and Bonding. Sometimes babies may cluster feed not just for nutritional reasons but also for comfort and closeness to their mother. As baby becomes more aware of their surroundings, they may seek more reassurance and security from their caregiver which translates into increased suckling and nuzzling with mum.

Look after yourself. Cluster feeding is highly demanding and while it rarely lasts more than a day or two, the disrupted sleep and constant call for your attention and energy can be draining. Be patient – it won't last for long (though it may feel like it) – and make sure you stay hydrated and eat well to support your own energy needs. Muster support so you can rest when possible and, if you have any concerns, seek help from a lactation consultant, breastfeeding support group or healthcare professional.

How to tell if your baby is getting enough milk

When you formula feed, you can tell to the millimetre how much milk your baby has consumed. Breastfeeding does not come with a handy measurement gauge but there are still lots of ways to know if baby is getting enough milk:

Your baby will feed with long rhythmic sucks, and you will hear them swallowing

Their cheeks will stay rounded out, not sucked in, as they feed.

Your baby is calm during feeding and comes off the breast themselves when they have had enough and appear content and satisfied after most feeds.

Breastfed babies often lose a little weight in the first week after birth, but this will be regained as your milk supply is established. Check with your health visitor if they are unsettled after feeding and don't appear to be gaining weight.

After the first few days, your baby should have at least 6 wet nappies a day, and after the first week your baby's dirty nappies should stop looking black and thick but have soft or even runny yellow poos. These can be quite explosive so always have spare clothes to change baby when necessary.

Some top tips

If your breasts are engorged with milk, it can be hard for your baby to latch on. Try to hand express a little milk first to reduce the engorgement.

When your baby opens their mouth big and wide, like a giant yawn, you can help by lightly compressing your breast, giving the nipple and areola a wedge shape more closely resembling your baby's mouth, so they latch onto a good mouthful.

Be aware of your baby's hunger cues – rooting, chewing on their fist, looking round for you. It is much easier to feed a baby who is becoming hungry than one that is in a full hunger meltdown. If your baby is agitated, try to comfort them first and when their breathing is more settled, then offer the breast.

6.   Winding

All babies get wind, which can give them tummy aches and lead to sick-up. The good news is breastfed babies typically get less wind and sick-up issues than formula babies. The bad news is they still get wind and sick-up issues. Winding or burping your baby is important to help them release any swallowed air during feeding and is something I wished I'd known more about with my first baby – by babies two and three I realised how important it was to help them expel any gas and remove discomfort:

Experiment with different winding positions to see which one is most effective for your baby. Some babies prefer being over the shoulder, while others may respond better to being seated on your lap. Some prefer being on their tummy, lying across your arm or knee as the pressure helps ease tummy pain.

Whichever position you pick, make sure baby's head is supported and in a neutral position and that they are comfortable and safe. Use gentle patting or rubbing motions on your baby's back, particularly in the mid-back area, between the shoulder blades. You can use your palm or fingertips. The patting should be firm but not forceful.

You can also help your baby release gas by lying them on their back and gently moving their legs in a bicycle-like motion.

You can burp your baby during and after a breastfeeding session. It's common to wind your baby when switching breasts if they haven't burped yet.

Not all babies will burp after every feed, and some may require more winding than others. Be patient and continue winding for a few minutes if needed. You will get to know your baby's habits over time.

Each baby is unique, so pay attention to your baby's cues and adjust your winding routine accordingly. If you have worries, and baby seems to be in acute pain after feeding, check in with your health visitor or paediatrician.

7.　　Breast pumps and more

In the modern world, a woman cannot be a 24/7 milk machine. This is where it can be so useful to express milk, which can be stored for those times when you need to be apart from your baby, whether for work, medical appointments or your own wellbeing. Expressed milk is also a great way for partners and other caregivers to enjoy the experience of feeding and building their own bond with baby.

Expressing milk is also a great way to increase your milk production, particularly in those early days when you're trying to establish supply – remember, the more milk you release, whether through feeding or pumping, the more your body will make.

It is possible to hand express small amounts of milk, but most women find it is far more efficient to use a breast pump. There are manual and electric pumps, and single and double pumps. Consider how often you plan to use the pump. If you'll be pumping frequently, a double electric pump is generally the most convenient choice. For occasional use, a manual or single electric pump may suffice.

Clearly, this is not the most glamourous purchase you are going to make but it can be very useful in ensuring breastfeeding success. Do some research into models and makes, and look on re-selling sites, like eBay, or local mum-and-toddler groups, as they are often sold or passed on second hand for a fraction of the cost of buying new (wash and sterilise thoroughly of course).

Find a quiet spot to pump, near an electric outlet if needed. You may find massaging and a warm compress applied to your breast can help to stimulate milk flow. Sometimes it can be difficult to get started, particularly if you're away from your baby – try to relax, think about your baby. Imagine them with you and you may find just the emotional connection even at a distance is enough to get the hormones doing their job.

Your flow may start off slow but don't worry – try to stay relaxed, be patient and make sure the pump is properly fitted over your breast to form a vacuum. After about ten minutes, you may be surprised how much milk has collected but keep going until your breasts feel soft and the milk is no longer flowing - emptying the breasts thoroughly helps maintain milk supply.

Store the milk in clean food-grade containers or breastmilk storage bags – just squeeze out the excess air before sealing. Be sure to label with the date so you know to use the oldest milk first. Store in small portions (2 to 4 ounces or 60-120 ml) to reduce waste - you can always combine multiple portions for a single feeding.

You can store freshly expressed breast milk in the refrigerator for up to 4-5 days at temperatures of 32-39°F (0-4°C). Make sure you store it in the back of the refrigerator, rather than the door, to maintain a consistent temperature.

You can also freeze breast milk, for up to 12 months. Freeze milk in small portions to make it easier to thaw and use only what your baby needs. Leave some space at the top of the container or bag to allow for milk expansion during freezing. To thaw the breast milk, move it to the refrigerator the night before you plan to use it or thaw it by putting the container or bag in a bowl of warm water. Once thawed, gently mix or stir the milk and use within 24 hours. Do not refreeze.

If your baby doesn't finish a bottle of breast milk, discard the remaining milk within 2 hours.

Keys, phone, purse…and pump

If you are going to be away from your baby for an extended period, missing several nursing sessions, be sure to take your breast pump with you. Otherwise, your breasts will become uncomfortably engorged and your milk supply may suffer. Some workplaces now set up quiet rooms where nursing mothers can express milk in private, and even have special locked fridges where the pumped milk can be stored – if this is your employer, give them a high five. Too many of us have experienced the indignity of having to pump milk in toilets with the expressed milk tipped down the sink because there was no place to store it safely. Fortunately, times are changing but it certainly helps to explain why breastfeeding rates remain stubbornly low in some societies.

8.   Out and about

While you recover from birth and spend time getting to know your newborn, you're likely to spend a lot of time at home. This nesting time is important to help you rest, rebuild your strength, bond with baby and establish a good feeding regime. But before too long you will be out and about to run errands, visit friends and family, attend medical appointments and introduce baby to the big wide world.

For many new mums, the thought of breastfeeding in public can be daunting, with fears of being judged for "doing it wrong", or for reasons of modesty and embarrassment. Try to relax, every new mother feels judged for everything at some point – human beings love to weigh in with helpful and unhelpful commentary which is generally best dealt with a polite nod and then forgotten about. And there is nothing to feel embarrassed about: you are feeding your baby in the most natural way. It is a biological function that ensured the success and survival of our species over millennia – be proud of what your body can do.

Even so, here are a few pointers to make your first outings more successful:

Know Your Rights. Familiarize yourself with the laws regarding breastfeeding in public in your area. In many places, it is legally protected, and you have the right to breastfeed wherever you and your baby are allowed to be.

Dress Comfortably. Wear clothing that allows for easy access to your breast, such as nursing tops, button-down shirts, or clothing with discreet openings. A nursing cover or shawl can also provide extra coverage if you prefer.

Practice at Home. If you're nervous about nursing in public, practice breastfeeding at home with a mirror to get a sense of how discreet you can be. Remember, depending on what you're wearing, your baby's head will cover most of your breast so while you may feel very exposed, in reality passersby probably won't see a thing.

Plan Ahead. Think about your baby's normal feeding schedule to either minimise the need for nursing in public if it makes you anxious, or to ensure you're in a comfortable feeding-friendly spot at baby's normal feed time. Research venues that are known to be breastfeeding-friendly, such as libraries, parks, or family-friendly restaurants. If you drive, you may find your own car parked in a discreet spot is most convenient for a feed and nappy change.

Anticipate and act. Notice when baby is signalling hunger and feed quickly to avert a meltdown that will draw attention to you. I certainly remember drawing the eye of everyone in a busy café when my baby had an ear-splitting hunger rage and worked himself up into such a state he couldn't feed despite my efforts to get him to latch on. It feels mortifying at the time but it's just life and the embarrassment soon fades.

Be polite but firm. Should anybody express disapproval, politely inform them of your legal right to breastfeed and emphasize the importance of normalizing breastfeeding in public. It's their problem, not yours. If it continues, try to remain calm and composed, and report the incident to the management of the venue if appropriate.

Safety in numbers. Join up with other breastfeeding mums in your area. It can provide emotional support and shared experiences.

Essentials

Going out and about with a breastfed baby means you don't need to think about spare formula, bottles, cool bags or bottle warmers. Have breast, then you're good go though you still might need these essentials:

- Spare nappies, wipes and bags
- Spare baby clothes. Two sets.
- Muslin cloths for spit up
- Shawl or scarf for modesty
- Water and snacks for you

9.　Twins or more

Congratulations on your babies. Yes, it is absolutely possible to breastfeed twins, or even triplets. Be ready, however, for the challenges ahead so you can take them confidently in your stride. Patience, persistence and an ability to go-with-the-flow yet also be very organised will be key strengths for the journey ahead.

Get help and advice. If you're expecting twins or more and plan to breastfeed, consider consulting with a lactation consultant before or shortly after birth. They can provide guidance and support tailored to your specific situation.

Start Early. If possible, initiate skin-to-skin and breastfeeding as soon as your babies are born. Early breastfeeding can help establish your milk supply and encourage your babies to latch.

Use a Nursing Pillow A nursing pillow, such as a twin breastfeeding pillow, can provide valuable support in positioning both babies comfortably for breastfeeding.

Alternate Breasts. When breastfeeding twins, you can alternate breasts during each feeding session to ensure both babies receive adequate milk. This helps stimulate milk production in both breasts.

Tandem Nursing. Tandem nursing means breastfeeding both babies at the same time. It can be efficient and save time. Positions like the double football hold or the cradle hold for one baby and the football hold for the other can be used.

Frequent Feedings. Twins may need to nurse more frequently than singletons. Be prepared for more frequent feedings, especially in the early weeks.

Supplementing. In some cases, supplementation with expressed breast milk or formula may be necessary, especially if your babies were born prematurely or have special medical needs. Consult with a healthcare provider or lactation consultant if you have concerns about milk supply.

Support Network. Enlist the help of a support network, including family and friends, to assist with chores and other responsibilities so you can focus on breastfeeding and caring for your twins.

Stay Hydrated, Eat Well and Rest. Proper nutrition, hydration and rest are important to support milk production, especially when breastfeeding two or more babies. Try to nap or rest when your babies are sleeping.

Pump if Necessary. A breast pump can help you maintain your milk supply and provide breast milk when you can't breastfeed directly. It can also be a great way to enlist helpers who can help bottle feed to give you a break.

Join a Support Group. Consider joining a breastfeeding support group for mothers of twins. It can be valuable to connect with others who have similar experiences.

10.　　Managing your toddler too

Keeping a toddler entertained while breastfeeding a newborn can be a juggling act but with some creativity and planning, it's possible to balance the needs of both children. Here are some strategies to keep your toddler entertained and help avoid jealousy:

Before baby arrives. Talk to your toddler about what to expect and help them be included in planning for the arrival of "baby brother/sister". Encourage them to be more independent in some activities, such as dressing themselves or picking out their snacks, but remember they are still little babies themselves and will need extra comfort and reassurance in the coming months.

Special Toddler Box. Create a special box of toys, books, and activities that your toddler can only access during breastfeeding sessions. This will make these items more enticing and make baby's breastfeeding a time to relish rather than resent. Puzzles, colouring and sticker books and building blocks can be great to encourage some quiet independent play.

Toddler-Friendly Snacks. Have a stash of healthy snacks that your toddler can enjoy during breastfeeding. This can help keep them occupied and satisfied but do keep an eye on them at all times.

Storytime. Read books to your toddler while you breastfeed. You can create a special reading corner near your nursing area for this purpose and it ensures your toddler gets to snuggle with you at the same time as baby.

Educational Apps or Videos. Realistically, in today's society we all use screens, be it TV or educational apps, to buy ourselves a little quiet time from our toddler's demands – and this can be useful while breastfeeding. And there's nothing wrong with this as long as the screentime is balanced by time playing with toys or exploring outside.

Involve Them. If your toddler is interested, involve them in caring for the baby. They can help with tasks like bringing diapers or choosing baby clothes. If they have a baby doll, they can be encouraged to mirror you and feed their doll as you feed baby.

Special bonding time. Set aside some one-on-one bonding time with your toddler during the day when the baby is asleep. This can help reassure them that they still hold a special place in your heart.

Routine and predictability. It can be chaotic and busy when a newborn arrives in the house but don't let that completely disrupt the routine that helps your toddler feel calm and in control. Try to establish a consistent daily routine that includes playtime, meals, and naps to help your toddler know what to expect.

Muster help. If possible, enlist the help of a partner, family member, or caregiver to spend quality time with your toddler while you focus on breastfeeding the baby. Make sure this time is a treat time for your toddler, so they don't feel pushed out.

Patience and understanding. It's perfectly normal for toddlers to have bouts of jealously and to even regress when a new baby arrives. It's a time that can throw up some big emotions for little people who don't yet have the emotional regulation or language to express themselves. Be patient and offer extra reassurance and love during these moments.

Help them find age-appropriate words to express how they feel and find outlets, through painting or outside play, to work off some negative energy. Help your toddler notice how baby is your toddlers biggest superfan and nurture a loving relationship that will be with them throughout their lives. In time, the two of them will be best of friends and running rings round you!

11.   Dealing with challenges

Sore nipples

It happens. This is a brand-new activity for you, and your nipples and tender breast skin need a bit of time to adjust. But there's a lot you can do to both avoid soreness and remedy it should it occur:

Ensure a Proper Latch. One of the most common causes of sore nipples is an improper latch. Make sure your baby is latching onto the breast correctly and taking a good mouthful of the areola (the dark area around the nipple) along with the nipple. Their lips should be flanged like a fish. Seek assistance from a lactation consultant or healthcare provider if you're unsure about the latch.

Vary Nursing Positions. Change nursing positions to reduce pressure on specific areas of the nipple. Experiment with different holds to find what works best for you and your baby.

Break the Suction Gently. After nursing, break the suction gently by inserting a clean finger into the corner of your baby's mouth and easing the latch before removing the breast.

Use Breast Milk. After nursing, express a few drops of breast milk and rub it onto your nipples. Breast milk has natural healing properties that can help soothe and protect sore nipples.

Nipple Creams/Balms. Apply lanolin-based nipple creams or ointments to your nipples before and after each feed to moisturize and provide relief.

Air Dry. Allow your nipples to air dry after each feed to promote healing and prevent moisture buildup, which can contribute to soreness. Having babies is a great cure for modesty – let it all hang out!

Use Breast Pads. Use breast pads to keep your clothing dry and prevent friction on sensitive nipples.

Pain Relief. Over-the-counter pain relievers, such as ibuprofen or paracetamol, can help alleviate pain and inflammation. Always check dosage and follow the instructions.

Seek Professional Help. If soreness persists or worsens, consult with a lactation consultant or healthcare provider. There may be an underlying issue that requires assessment and treatment, such as thrush or a tongue tie.

Mastitis

Mastitis is an inflammatory condition of the breast tissue that can cause pain, swelling, redness, and warmth in one or both breasts. It can develop when the breast becomes engorged due to milk buildup and is not adequately drained or if a milk duct becomes blocked with milk. This can occur when the baby does not feed frequently or effectively. Cracked or sore nipples can create an entry point for bacteria, increasing the risk of infection.

The symptoms of mastitis can vary but often include:

- Breast pain and tenderness, often localized to one area.
- Redness, swelling, or warmth in the affected breast.
- A hard lump or wedge-shaped area of the breast.
- Fever and chills.
- Flu-like symptoms, such as fatigue and body aches.
- Nipple discharge containing blood or pus.

Mastitis should be promptly treated to prevent complications.

Seek medical attention and follow these tips:

Continue Breastfeeding. It's crucial to continue breastfeeding from the affected breast to help clear the infection. The baby's sucking can help drain the breast so feed more frequently from the affected breast and start feeds with the affected breast and change positions to help drain different areas. If breastfeeding is too painful, you can express milk using a breast pump to maintain milk supply and prevent further engorgement.

Heat Compress. Applying a warm compress to the affected area before feeding can help reduce pain and encourage milk flow.

Pain Relief. Over-the-counter pain relievers like ibuprofen or paracetamol can help reduce pain and inflammation.

Rest and Hydration. Get plenty of rest and stay well-hydrated to support your body's healing process.

Antibiotics. Your healthcare provider may prescribe antibiotics to clear the infection. Make sure you finish the course.

C-Section

Breastfeeding after a C-section may come with some unique challenges due to the surgery and recovery process. But many women still successfully breastfeed after a C-Section, me included! Here are some top tips to help you have a successful breastfeeding experience after a C-section:

Start Early. Even in the operating theatre, it's possible to begin skin-to-skin. This can be continued in the recovery room, when baby may do the milk crawl to initiate suckling, or your partner or midwife can help position baby.

Pillows and positions. A nursing pillow can help position your baby comfortably and take pressure off your incision. Some useful positions are side-lying position and football hold. Use pillows in cradle hold to ensure there's no pressure on your incision.

Pain Management. Take prescribed pain medications to manage pain and discomfort from the C-section. Pain can hinder your ability to nurse comfortably, so staying on top of it is important.

Keep Baby Close. Your mobility may be limited at first to make sure you have help.

Stay Hydrated and Nourished. Drink plenty of water and eat nutritious meals to support your milk production and energy levels.

Rest and Recover. Ensure you're getting adequate rest and sleep to support your physical and emotional well-being, which can impact milk production.

Use a Breast Pump. If you're having trouble with latching or your milk supply, consider using a breast pump to express milk and feed your baby. Pumping can help maintain your milk supply until your baby can nurse effectively.

Allergies

Breast milk is considered one of the most hypoallergenic and easily digestible sources of nutrition for infants. However, some babies may have allergies or sensitivities to certain proteins or substances that are passed into breast milk from the mother's diet. If you think this is the case, consult with your healthcare provider for advice.

Cow's Milk Protein Allergy (CMPA). Some babies may be sensitive or allergic to proteins found in cow's milk. If a breastfeeding mother consumes dairy products, these proteins can pass into her breast milk and potentially cause symptoms in the baby, such as colic, eczema, diarrhoea, or fussiness. In such cases, a healthcare provider may recommend eliminating dairy from the mother's diet.

Other Food Allergies or Sensitivities. Babies can also react to other foods that the mother consumes. Common culprits include soy, nuts, wheat, and eggs. Symptoms in the baby may include fussiness, skin rashes, or digestive issues. Eliminating the suspected allergen from the mother's diet can help alleviate symptoms.

Medications. Certain medications or supplements that a mother takes can potentially pass into breast milk and affect the baby. It's essential for breastfeeding mothers to consult with their doctor or pharmacist about the safety of any medications or supplements.

Environmental Allergens. Babies can also be exposed to environmental allergens through breast milk if the mother is exposed to them. However, this is less common and usually related to allergens such as pollen or pet dander.

Dealing with illness

Babies can continue to breastfeed when they are unwell. Indeed, breastfeeding is often beneficial for an unwell baby – it's easily digestible and contains antibodies, enzymes, and immune cells that can help the baby's immune system fight off infections and provides hydration and comfort, which are especially important when a baby is unwell.

Offer frequent breastfeeds. Sick babies may have reduced appetite and may not feed as vigorously as usual so offer your breast more frequently to ensure they get enough nutrition and hydration.

Monitor hydration. Pay attention to signs of dehydration, such as fewer wet nappies, dry mouth, or sunken soft spots on the baby's head. Breast milk is an excellent source of hydration for sick infants. Adjust feeding positions: Depending on the baby's illness, they may be more comfortable in certain feeding positions. Experiment with different breastfeeding positions to find one that works best for both you and your baby.

Nasal congestion. If the baby has nasal congestion, you can use a saline nasal spray or drops to clear their nasal passages before feeding. Always check with a healthcare professional first and follow the instructions.

Consult a doctor. If your baby's illness is severe, accompanied by difficulty breathing, or involves specific symptoms that concern you, seek immediate medical attention. Your healthcare provider can offer advice on how to manage breastfeeding during serious illnesses.

Tongue tie

A tongue tie (ankyloglossia) is when the thin piece of tissue (the lingual frenulum) beneath the baby's tongue is shorter than usual, restricting the tongue's range of motion. This can interfere with the baby's ability to latch onto the breast, create a good seal and effectively remove milk from the breast.

The impact of a tongue tie on breastfeeding can vary from mild to severe, and not all babies with tongue ties will experience significant breastfeeding difficulties. Two of my babies had tongue-ties, one lost interest in breastfeeding before six months because he was finding it hard work and much preferred to be bottle-fed but the other, despite some initial nipple discomfort for me, successfully fed for almost two years.

Some common issues are:
Shallow latch. The baby may have difficulty latching deeply onto the breast, leading to nipple pain and damage.

Ineffective milk transfer. A restricted tongue movement can make it challenging for the baby to create enough suction to effectively remove milk from the breast. This can then signal the body to produce less milk, potentially leading to low milk supply.

Fussiness and frustration. Babies with tongue ties may become frustrated during feeds, as they are unable to effectively extract milk.

Slow weight gain. In some cases, babies with severe tongue ties may experience slow weight gain due to inadequate milk intake. Consult with your healthcare provider; if breastfeeding is to persist, you may need to pump breastmilk and supplement with expressed milk or formula to ensure baby is getting enough nourishment.

The decision to address a tongue tie depends on the severity of breastfeeding difficulties and the impact on both the baby and mother. Some tongue ties may improve naturally as the baby grows, while others may require intervention. The most common treatment for tongue tie is a simple procedure called a frenotomy or frenuloplasty, where a healthcare provider clips or releases the tight band of tissue under the baby's tongue.

Consult with your healthcare provider about the best options and talk to a lactation consultant about potential tongue-tie friendly positions and techniques.

Inverted nipples

If your nipples are inverted, breastfeeding may take some more effort but it's still possible. Consult a lactation consultant for specialist advice. Breast pumping may help, or you could try a nipple shield. This is a thin soft, flexible silicone device that's worn over your nipple and has small holes in the tip that allow the milk to flow into your baby's mouth and which may help guide your baby to latch on more deeply if other interventions aren't working.

Breast refusal

When baby refuses to feed from one breast, it can be challenging, with the neglected breast becoming engorged and, potentially, impacting supply. Babies can develop a preference for one breast over the other due to factors like milk flow, breast shape, or nipple size.

Here are some tips:

Check for Latching Issues. Ensure that your baby is latching correctly. A poor latch or discomfort during nursing can lead to a baby refusing one breast. Seek help from a lactation consultant or healthcare provider to assess and improve the latch.

Examine the Breast. Inspect the breast your baby is refusing. Look for signs of soreness, redness, or a blocked milk duct. Any pain or discomfort on that breast can lead to rejection. You may need to address issues like mastitis or nipple thrush.

Breast Milk Supply. Evaluate your milk supply. If your baby is frustrated because the milk is flowing too slowly, you can try breast compressions or massage to encourage milk flow on the less preferred side. Make sure both breasts are being adequately emptied during feeds.

Switch Nursing. Try "switch nursing," where you switch sides several times during a single feeding session. This can help ensure both breasts are fully drained, and your baby gets the hindmilk (fattier milk) on both sides.

Offer During Sleep. Some babies may be more willing to nurse from the less preferred breast while drowsy or sleepy. Try offering the breast during your baby's sleepy moments.

Pump the Refused Breast. To maintain milk supply, pump the breast that your baby is refusing to nurse from. You can then offer this expressed milk to your baby in a bottle or cup.

Distraction

Babies can become easily distracted during breastfeeding, especially as they grow and become more aware of their surroundings. Here are some strategies to help your baby stay focused on breastfeeding:

Choose a Quiet Environment. Find a quiet, calm place to breastfeed. Dim the lights and minimize noise and distractions, such as the TV or phone, which might grab your baby's attention. When out and about, a lightweight blanket or shawl draped over your shoulder can help create a breastfeeding "cocoon" for your baby.

Swaddle. Swaddling your baby before feeding can help create a cozy, comforting environment and reduce the distraction of their own limbs.

Burp Before Feeding. If your baby seems gassy or fussy, try burping them before starting a breastfeeding session. A burp can relieve discomfort and make it easier for your baby to focus on feeding.

Use a Nursing Necklace. Some babies enjoy playing with a nursing necklace (a safe, baby-friendly necklace) while breastfeeding, which can help keep them engaged with the task at hand.

Be patient. The world is exciting and new to your baby, and it's normal they want to learn about it. As your baby grows and matures, they may become better at managing distractions during feeds.

When it doesn't work

Sometimes breastfeeding just doesn't work out. Your milk supply may not come in, or baby may prefer the bottle or breastfeeding may prove incompatible with the realities of your busy life. And that's all OK. Do not beat yourself up.

I had a friend who exhausted herself with stress and worry as her baby's weight dropped sharply because she was determined to breastfeed come what may – but there wasn't enough milk and baby was failing to thrive. Fortunately, her mother – who had bottle-fed a brood of kids in the 1970s – came to visit and took one look at the baby, ran to the shops to buy bottles and formula and the baby quickly regained weight. My friend, however, used to hide the bottles when her breastfeeding friends came round, such was the stigma she felt at having "failed" at breastfeeding. Yet her baby has no memories of this and having grown into a healthy headstrong and talented university student, is the very definition of successful parenting.

What matters is a healthy baby, and a healthy mum. No baby remembers how they were fed – all that matters is they got the nourishment they needed to grow and develop, and the love and attention to feel safe and secure in this big new world.

Repeat to yourself: it does not matter. Bottle or breast, it's all good. Your baby loves you regardless of feeding method so let go of the guilt and focus on the little human being in your life. These precious days go by fast so focus on making the most of them. Let it go and move forward with love and joy.

For more advice on bottle-feeding, be sure to read our newborn survival guide, Everyday Expertise: New Baby

12.   Your health

Your baby needs you to stay fit and well, both physically, mentally and emotionally. Looking after yourself is part of looking after baby so make sure you take care of your own wellbeing: motherhood is not another word for martyr!

Here are important considerations regarding nutrition, health, diet, and alcohol for nursing mothers:

Nutrition Calorie Intake. According to the American College of Obstetricians and Gynaecologists, your body needs about 450 to 500 extra calories a day to make breast milk for your baby[4]. You may find you crave sugary foods but try to eat a healthy well-balanced diet with plenty of fruits, vegetables, lean proteins, whole grains and healthy fats. Avoid eating fish with high mercury levels – limit albacore tuna to 6 ounces a week.

Hydration. Staying well-hydrated is essential for milk production. Drink plenty of water throughout the day – use a re-usable water bottle and keep it handy to stay topped up with fluids on the go.

Nutrition. Ensure you're getting enough calcium to support your bone health from dairy products, fortified plant-based milks, leafy greens, and calcium supplements. Iron needs are increased during lactation so think about iron-rich foods like lean meats, beans, lentils, and fortified cereals. Omega-3s, found in fatty fish, flaxseeds, and walnuts, are crucial for infant brain development so try to incorporate these in your diet.

Folate. Continue taking prenatal vitamins or supplements that contain folate to support your own health.

Caffeine. You can consume moderate amounts of caffeine (about 200 mg a day) while breastfeeding, but excessive caffeine intake may lead to irritability and sleep disturbances in your baby.

Alcohol. If you choose to consume alcohol while breastfeeding, wait two hours after having a drink before breastfeeding to allow your body time to metabolize it. Pumping and storing milk in advance can also be an option if you plan to have a drink. Make sure that you are sober and alert when caring for your baby, especially during nighttime feedings or if you will be the sole caregiver.

Smoking and drug use. Smoking isn't good for you, and it isn't good for your baby, with second-hand smoking a known risk factor in sudden infant death syndrome. Using illegal drugs or misusing prescription drugs can harm your baby when breastfeeding as well as the risks to the baby should you become drowsy or incapacitated as a result of your drug use.

If you need help to quit smoking or drugs, there is no better time than now to reach out to your health visitor, doctor or support network. You can do this, for you and your baby.

Medications. Inform your healthcare provider that you are breastfeeding to ensure any medications prescribed are safe for nursing mothers and their infants.

Vaccinations. Check with your healthcare provider to ensure that you are up to date on vaccines, as some vaccines are recommended for breastfeeding mothers.

When mum is ill

In many cases, a baby can continue to breastfeed as it provides the baby with antibodies and immune-boosting factors that can help protect the baby from getting sick or reduce the severity of the illness if they do get sick.

Keep feeding. The majority of common illnesses, such as colds, flu, and mild infections, are not transmitted through breast milk. Instead, they are typically transmitted through respiratory droplets or direct contact. Therefore, breastfeeding is usually safe even when the mother is unwell with these types of illnesses.

Hand Hygiene and Respiratory Etiquette. To minimize the risk of transmitting illness to the baby, however, it's important to practice good hand hygiene and respiratory etiquette (covering the mouth and nose when coughing or sneezing, or even wearing a face mask while unwell).

Rest and Self-Care. It's crucial for the mother to prioritize her own health and recovery when she's unwell. Getting adequate rest, staying hydrated, and following any prescribed treatments or medications are important steps to facilitate her own healing and well-being. Make sure your doctor knows you are breastfeeding so that any medications are safe for nursing infants.

Temporary Reduction in Milk Supply. Some illnesses or medications may temporarily affect milk supply, but this is often reversible once the mother recovers. Frequent breastfeeding or pumping can help maintain milk supply during illness.

In rare cases, there may be circumstances where it is not advisable for a mother to breastfeed due to a severe illness, at which point healthcare providers can provide guidance on appropriate alternatives, such as expressed breast milk, donor milk, or formula feeding.

Your emotional health

Your body has been through a huge transition – pregnancy, labour and now breastfeeding. In addition to the physical changes, including the hormones flooding your system to support these different life stages, motherhood brings many mental and emotional challenges – you may find yourself tearful, anxious, self-questioning, exhausted and low. You may question your identity or find yourself at odds with your partner or other family members.

This is all normal and it's important to be kind to yourself – this is a stage of life that will pass and one day you will look back and be amazed at what you achieved. It is OK not to feel OK.

If you feel overwhelmed, speak to someone – whether it's your partner, your health visitor or your friends.

Make time for yourself, to connect with people and activities that were important to you before baby came along.

Try to get outside every day, even if it's just for a short walk and stretch in the sunshine.

You are still you, even if you do now have a mini-you alongside you on this journey called life. Be kind to yourself.

13.   Weaning

The time will come when it's time to weaning your baby off breast milk. This can be a significant transition for both of you, so take it slowly and carefully.

Timing is Personal. The timing of weaning varies from one mother and baby pair to another. It's a decision that should be based on what works best for both you and your baby. The WHO recommends continuing breastfeeding for up to two years or longer – alongside solid foods – but in reality, many mothers and babies stop before then. It is up to you.

Pay attention to baby's cues. Watch for signs that your baby is ready to wean. Some babies lose interest in breastfeeding as they become more interested in solid foods or other forms of nourishment.

Take it slow. Gradual weaning is generally recommended to minimize discomfort from engorgement and emotional distress for the baby. Start by eliminating one breastfeeding session per day and replacing it with a suitable alternative. It may be that your partner steps in with a bottle-feed for the dropped nursing session so the link between you and food/comfort is gradually broken. Continue this process over a period of several weeks or months until all feedings are replaced.

Offer Alternatives. When weaning, introduce appropriate alternatives to breast milk, such as formula, expressed breast milk, or solid foods, depending on the baby's age and readiness. You can gradually replace breastfeeding sessions with these alternatives.

Comfort and emotional support. Weaning can be an emotional process for both the baby and the mother. Be prepared to offer extra comfort, cuddling, and reassurance to your baby during this time.

Engorgement and pain. As you reduce breastfeeding sessions, you may experience breast engorgement and discomfort. Ease down slowly and use cold compresses or over-the-counter pain relievers if needed. It's important not to stimulate the breasts to produce more milk during this time or you will be locked in a cycle of milk production.

Patience is Key. Remember that every baby is different, and the weaning process can take time. Be patient with your baby and yourself, and don't rush the process.

Maintain Bonding. Even as you wean, continue to bond with your baby through cuddling, eye contact, and skin-to-skin contact. The emotional connection established during breastfeeding can be maintained in other ways.

References

[1] US Department of Health & Human Services, Breastfeeding: Surgeon General's Call to Action Fact Sheet
www.hhs.gov/surgeongeneral/reports-and-publications/breastfeeding/factsheet/index.html

[2] Both the World Health Organization (WHO) and the American Academy of Pediatrics (AAP) recommend exclusive breastfeeding for the first six months, without any water, formula, or solid foods.

[3] World Health Organization, Breastfeeding
www.who.int/news-room/questions-and-answers/item/breastfeeding

[4] American College of Obstetricians and Gynecologists, Breastfeeding Your Baby
www.acog.org/womens-health/faqs/Breastfeeding-Your-Baby?utm_source=redirect&utm_medium=web&utm_campaign=otn

More Everyday Expertise

If you found this book helpful, you may also want to read some of our other bite-sized Everyday Expertise guides.

Visit our website **www.everydayexpertise.net**

About Everyday Expertise

Founded by author and journalist Amy McLellan, Everyday Expertise publishes bite-size books on everyday topics to help make life better. From childcare and parenting to finances and health, our books are written and edited by teams of experts to deliver trusted insight and advice to help you navigate life, build healthier habits and make smarter decisions. Our books are short, affordable and advocate a common-sense approach. Making life better, one day at a time.

Disclaimer

Everyday Expertise's editors and writers are not medical professionals. We provide insight and advice based on the latest scientific research, the public guidance of medical associations and our own personal experiences. Our books are intended to inform your own decision-making process and Everyday Expertise has no responsibility for any damages, direct or indirect, arising from following any of published material. If you or anyone in your care has a physical or mental health issue, please consult a medical professional.